Essential Oils

A GUIDE FOR USING AROMATHERAPY IN YOUR EVERYDAY LIFE

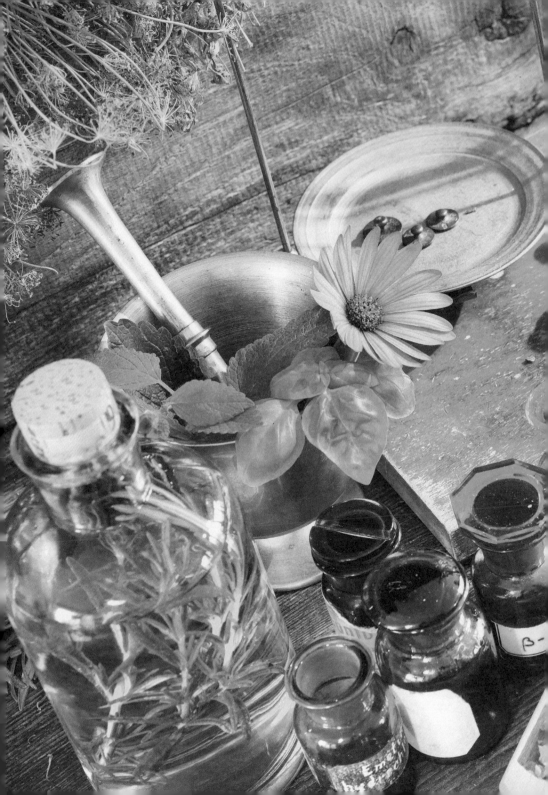

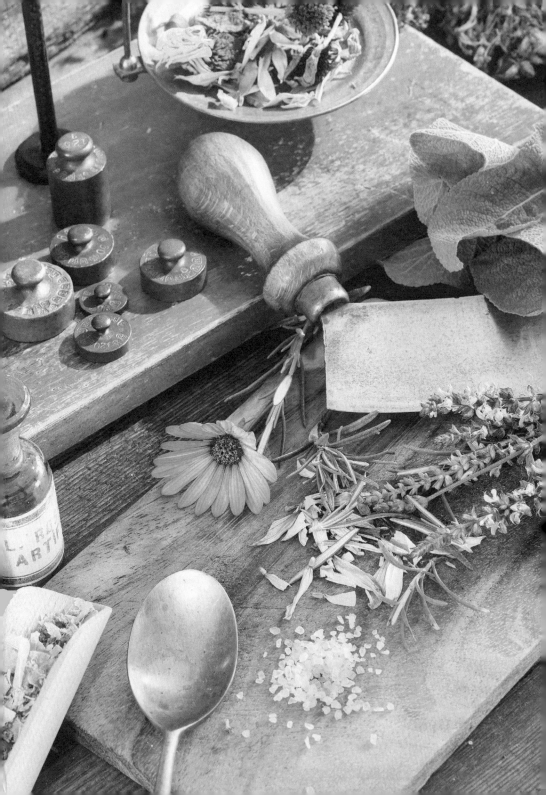

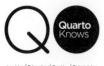

Inspiring | Educating | Creating | Entertaining

Brimming with creative inspiration, how-to projects, and useful information to enrich your everyday life, Quarto Knows is a favorite destination for those pursuing their interests and passions. Visit our site and dig deeper with our books into your area of interest: Quarto Creates, Quarto Cooks, Quarto Homes, Quarto Lives, Quarto Drives, Quarto Explores, Quarto Gifts, or Quarto Kids.

First published in 2016 by Wellfleet Press, an imprint of The Quarto Group, 142 West 36th Street, 4th Floor, New York, NY 10018, USA
T (212) 779-4972 F (212) 779-6058 **www.QuartoKnows.com**

Wellfleet titles are also available at discount for retail, wholesale, promotional, and bulk purchase. For details, contact the Special Sales Manager by email at specialsales@quarto.com or by mail at The Quarto Group, Attn: Special Sales Manager, 100 Cummings Center Suite 265D, Beverly, MA 01915 USA.

10 9 8 7 6 5 4 3 2 1

ISBN: 978-1-57715-221-7

Editorial Director: Francine LaSala
Author: Iside Sarmiento
Photo Credits: page 119
Project Editor: Karen Matsu Greenberg, Hourglass Press
Designer: Keira McGuinness

Printed in Singapore COS122019

This book provides general information. It should not be relied upon as recommending or promoting any specific diagnosis or method of treatment for a particular condition, and it is not intended as a substitute for medical advice or for direct diagnosis and treatment of a medical condition by a qualified physician. Readers who have questions about a particular condition, possible treatments for that condition, or possible reactions from the condition or its treatment should consult a physician or other qualified healthcare professional.

Essential Oils

A GUIDE FOR USING AROMATHERAPY
IN YOUR EVERYDAY LIFE

ISIDE SARMIENTO

WELLFLEET
PRESS

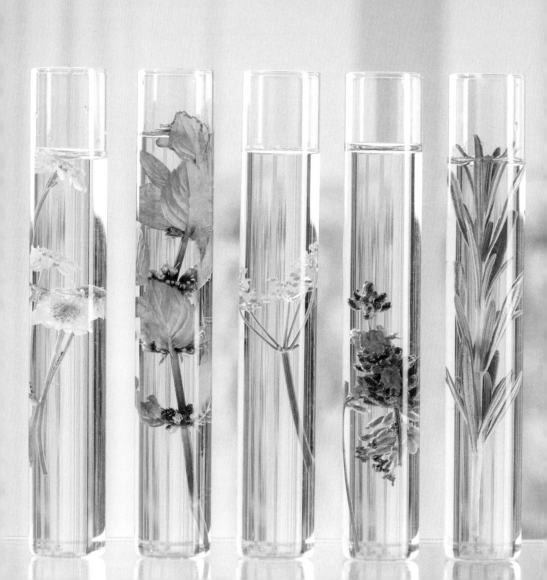

Contents

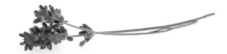

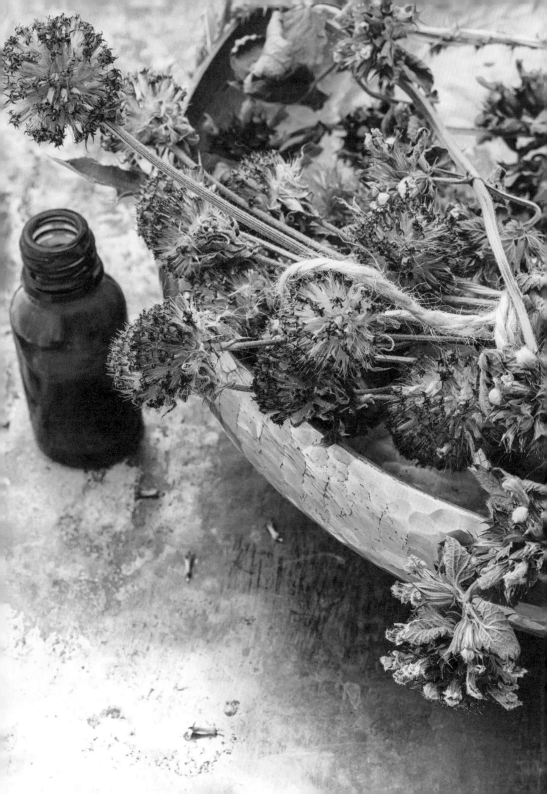

Author's Note

Inhale. Feel your atoms expanding and your sense of well-being improving as you breathe. You are starting to feel more alert.

Breathing keeps us alive, but it also keeps us vibrant. Sadly, the older we get, the less we breathe. Babies up to six weeks inhale thirty to sixty breaths per minute. They are literally absorbing life in every breath they take. Middle-aged adults only take twelve to eighteen breaths per minute, and the elderly, only ten breaths a minute. In addition to oxygenating our blood, breathing also helps us create memories. We breathe in the moment and make it last. But if we are breathing less are we also remembering less?

Aromatherapy is about using essential oils to help balance our bodies and minds, whether we are breathing them in, applying them, or even tasting them. It's about the power of scent to keep us regulated. The difference between herbs and essential oils is that essential oils are seventy to eighty times more powerful and concentrated than herbs and they work faster. One single drop of strong therapeutic-grade peppermint essential oil is comparable to drinking twenty-seven cups of peppermint-leaf tea.

If you have trouble sleeping at night because you suffer from "thinking overload," a little lavender scent in your pillow can help relieve those restless nights. If you have a headache, you can apply a drop of high-quality organic peppermint oil to your temples and within minutes, 90 percent of the time, the headache will disappear. Nauseated? Add ginger and peppermint oils to sparking water. It is refreshing and also calms the stomach.

Emotions are very diverse, and most individuals will experience more than one emotion at any given time. The best oils to motivate and encourage are: coriander, melissa, basil, rosemary, tangerine, and vanilla. The best oils to cheer or uplift the spirit are lemon, orange, ginger, and cinnamon. For peace and reassurance use lavender, vetiver, ylang ylang, frankincense, clary sage, marjoram, and spearmint.

When using an essential oil topically, proceed with caution. Do a patch test, perhaps on the sole of your foot. Also, always avoid the eyes. Even some very noble oils like lavender can cause an irritation or eruption in the skin. Some of the most potentially irritating to the skin oils include bergamot, birch, cassia, cinnamon, clove, lemongrass, oregano, peppermint, rosemary, wintergreen, and ylang-ylang.

When using essential oils internally, the first thing you need to be sure about is that they are pure and non-diluted or chemical-based essential oils. The ideal essential oils for ingestion are the ones mark as "Certified Pure Therapeutic Grade." Add these oils to your drinking water. Apply them under your tongue to stimulate digestion before meals or to alleviate gas, bloating, and spastic irritation.

Bear in mind that when ingesting essential oils, the more is not the merrier. A couple of drops a couple of times day is a great place to start. Your body weight, size, age, medications, usage experience, personality, and history are all factors to consider in using essential oils, as well as if you are pregnant. Pregnant women **need to be very careful** with how they use essential oils and which essential oils they use, as some may have adverse affects on the pregnancy, and some are not recommended to use at all.

However you use them, the benefits of essential oils far outweigh the drawbacks. No wonder aromatherapy has been around for thousands of years!

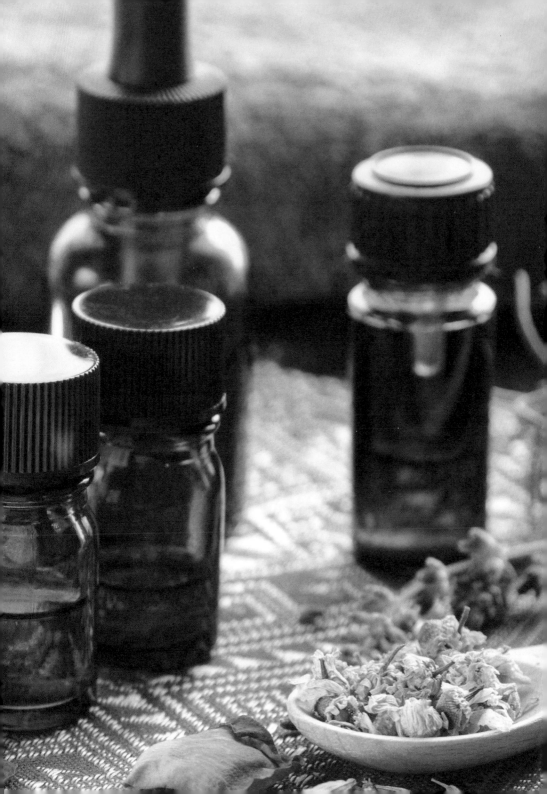

Introduction

Welcome to the exciting world of aromatherapy, the use of essential oils to essentially improve the quality of your life. With aromatherapy, you can become healthier by using combinations of these oils to actually create harmony in your life, not only by breathing them but also by using them topically and sometimes even by ingesting them. Additionally, you can use these as natural alternatives to beauty treatments, household cleansers, and air fresheners, and in other ways to allow you to enhance your overall sense of well-being.

Aromatherapy is "pure chemistry." It is "pure" because it relies on 100 percent pure essential oils — naturally extracted aromatic essences from plants; it's "chemistry" because the combinations of these oils create such a magical effect.

This book contains everything you need to get started to lead a more balanced life through aromatherapy, including information about essential oils and recipes for combining them to match so many occasions and needs.

Divided into four sections—About Aromatherapy, Carrier Oils, Essential Oils, and, finally, Recipes—this book will provide you with a firm foundation in the art of aromatherapy, and even inspire you to create your own recipes using essential oils.

Are you ready to start experiencing "better living through pure chemistry?" Good. Let's begin.

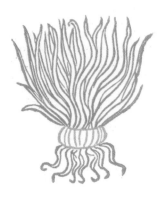

About Aromatherapy

Aromatherapy really started to come on the scene in the West in the early twentieth century, but aromatherapy has been used to promote health and well-being for thousands of years.

The ancient Egyptians burned incense as a way to honor their gods for more than 3,000 years B.C. They also embalmed and mummified their dead using aromatics, including frankincense and myrrh. Later, they would begin using aromatics for perfumes, cosmetics, and even medicine. King Tutankhamen used a valerian-based balsam for its calming properties, and the balm was found in its burial site with the rest of the treasures, still fragrant, when the tomb was opened in 1922.

The ancient Greeks were also big on aromatics, stating with the first physician Asclepius, who healed both through surgery and herbal remedies. Hippocrates, who also took a more holistic approach to medicine, later noted that "the

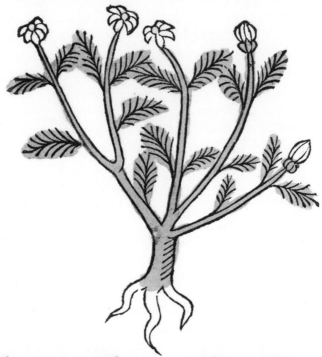

Camomilla   Camillen

Camomilla est calida ז sicca in primo. habet virtutē
mollificandi et dissoluendi. frondes et flores sunt eq̄
lis virtutis. Et aqua decoctōnis ei⁹ cū arthimesia cū
qua fomentetur matrix valz puocando menstruum
Idem valet mulieribus difficulter parientibꝰ. Deco
ctio floꝛ camomillaꝛ et extremitatū absinthei ז ra
vicū feniculi petrosilini ז quatuoꝛ seminum frigidoꝛ
in vino cū zucro albo dulcoꝛando de quo bibat̄ valz

key to good health rests on having a daily aromatic bath and scented massage."

It didn't stop there. A student of Aristotle, Theophrastus of Athens, published extensively about herbs and healing, while military physician Dioscorides put together *De Materia Medica*. The physician Claudius Galen treated the gladiators with medicinal herbs, and it is said that not a single gladiator died of battle wounds in his care.

When Rome fell, the use of aromatics as medicine in the Western world followed suit. But in the East, it continued to thrive. Persian physicians including Al-Razi and Ibn Sina booth incorporated aromatics as part of their practice. Ali-Ibn Sana wrote books on the properties of eight hundred

(opposite page) Chamomile, in *Herbarius Latinus,* from the press of Johann Petri at Passau, 1485. Courtesy of The National Library of Medicine.

plants and their effects on the human body, and is credited for being the first person to discover and record the method of distilling essential oils. His methods are still in use.

The Crusades helped bring it back to Western awareness, but because of the teachings of beliefs of the Catholic church and other controlling influences, it didn't thrive as it once had.

In fact, it wasn't until the twentieth century that the West began taking aromatics seriously again. The term *aromatherapie* was coined by a French chemist named René-Maurice Gattefossé in the 1920s. He worked in his family's perfume business and "discovered" the healing ability of lavender by accident when he burned his hand in a chemical accident and plunged it into a container of pure lavender oil. Following his discovery, more French chemists continued the study of aromatics and health for decades. Then, in 1977, *The Art of Aromatherapy* was published, the first aromatherapy book in English, and has essentially become the "bible" for aromatherapy.

In in the last five years, there has been a "boom" in the use of essential oils. Before 1950, there where about five publications on essential oils. By 1993, that number had grown to two hundred. By 2007, that number tripled to

René-Maurice Gattefossé

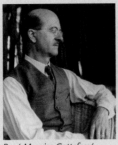
René-Maurice Gattefossé

Known as the Father of Aromatherapy, René-Maurice Gattefossé was born in 1881 in Montchat, France, and worked in his family's cosmetics factory. During an accident in the laboratory one day, he received a bad burn on his hand. Frantically looking around for liquid, he plunged his hand into the nearest tub of lavender essential oil. Amazed at how quickly his burn healed without scarring, he began to experiment with essential oils on wounded World War I soldiers. He first used lavender, thyme, lemon, and clove for their antiseptic qualities and noticed a high rate of healing with essential oils. Gattefossé wrote several books on essential oils, but his 1937 *Aromathérapie: Les Huiles Essentielles Hormones Végétales* is his legacy. After being translated to English as *Aromatherapy*, the rest, as they say, is history, and a name was born.

around six hundred; and nearly doubled again to more than a thousand in 2011. By 2013, there were over thirteen hundred publications about aromatherapy.

All of this is to say that aromatherapy is not just some new fad—it's a time-tested way to improve physical, mental, and emotional well-being.

What Exactly Is Aromatherapy?

Aromatherapy is a method of healing that calls on the use of aromatic essential oils. Aromatherapy works through inhalation, topical application, and ingestion— meaning that these oils can be inhaled, applied to the skin, and sometimes even swallowed. The essential oils are sometimes used in combination with one another and also added to "carrier" or "base" oils to achieve the desired effect.

Sometimes aromatherapy is used to treat an existing condition, but it can also be used in prevention. As you will see in the next section, many of the essential oils have properties that can boost immunity. And it's not just about physical health and well-being. Aromatherapy is also used to ease depression and anxiety; to enhance moods; and even to increase libido and improve sexual dysfunction.

Using essential oils in healing and maintaining well-being is generally safe, although there are some instances where allergies come into play. One way to limit allergic reaction is to make sure you use only genuine 100 percent essential oils in aromatherapy. You want to avoid using synthetic oils as you can't be entirely sure what you're getting. Always use glass containers or PET plastic (recyclable and food-safe) to mix and carry your oils.

How Does it Work?

Of all your senses, your sense of smell actually has the most direct connection to your mind, and all that your mind controls. Can you recall being a child, peeling that fresh orange during that super hot summer and how the scent when you smell it even now reminds you of summer? Or maybe a time when you were sick as a child and the fragrance of eucalyptus that gave you relief and a better night's sleep?

When you inhale aromatics, the scent stimulates olfactory receptor sites and sends messages to the limbic area of your brain, known as the rhinocephalon. Here, thirty-four structures and fifty-three pathways interpret the stimulus and, in turn, alert the areas for which the messages are intended. Aromatics can be inhaled using many methods, including diffusers, candles, and aromatic baths—which is also a boon for the skin.

Applying aromatics is usually done through some kind of massage, although they can also be applied directly to areas of the skin requiring aid, such in the case of cuts or burns. You can add essential oils to products you already use, and you can also check labels for things like shampoos, conditioners, moisturizers, and more. You may be surprised to see how often these aromatics come up.

Diffusers

There are many different types of diffusers available on the market, but all of them fall into one of four categories based on how they place the essential oil into the air: (1) nebulizing, (2) ultrasonic, or humidifying, (3) evaporative, and (4) heat. Each one has its own pros and cons.

Nebulizing diffusers, or nebulizers, are similar to perfume atomizers in which a jet of air blows oil into a fine spray or mist. Because nebulizers use the whole essential oil, it is considered the best and most powerful type of diffuser, as it will quickly saturate the air in a room. The cons are that they can be a bit noisier than other types of diffusers and also consume more oil.

Ultrasonic, or humidifying, diffusers also create a fine mist, like nebulizers, but use electronic frequencies and ultrasonic vibrations to disperse the essential oil into microparticles. Unlike nebulizers, ultrasonic diffusers only use a fraction of the oil and rely on a room's air current to disperse the mist, which make them perfect for those who want only a small amount of oil to be diffused.

Some evaporative diffusers use a fan to blow air from the room through a filter containing essential oil, while other types—which tend to be personal diffusers such as pendants, bracelets, or sachets—use the existing air current to distribute the oil. Although great for maintaining an aroma in small or personal spaces and being pretty quiet, this type of diffuser may diminish any therapeutic properties of the essential oil. This is because oils separate into lighter and heavier components when they evaporate. The lighter components evaporate more quickly and early in the process while the heavier components evaporate toward the end.

Heat diffusers are similar to evaporative diffusers in that they evaporate the essential oil more quickly than normal but use heat, instead of blowing air. Better heat diffusers only use low levels of heat that produce subtle aromas, which is preferred because high heat can alter the chemical makeup of the oil. Like all evaporation methods, you run the risk of fractioning the oil into components; on the other hand, they are completely quiet.

How Are Essential Oils Extracted?

Sometimes plants store oils externally and sometimes they are stored internally. When they are external, such as is with plants like basil, lavender, and mints, all you need to do to get to the aroma is to touch the plant. When they are internal, for example, in citruses, eucalyptus, and clove, you have to break the leaf or seed in order to get to the scent.

There are four methods used to remove oils from plants: (1) distillation, (2) expression, (3) solvent extraction, and, newer than the others, (4) hypercritical carbon dioxide (CO_2) extraction.

Distillation is the oldest method. Using water, steam, a combination of water and steam, or percolation, oils are extracted from plants where the oils are located externally. Water distillation is generally done with flowers, while a combination of water and steam is generally used with herbs and leaves. Steam on its own is used when higher temperatures are needed to extract the oils. With percolation, the steam comes through the top, rather than through the bottom, which speeds up the process, especially in the case of extracting oils from "woody" materials like fennel and dill.

Expression is also known as "cold pressing." It is used when the oils are internal. Here, the zest from the citrus is soaked first. Then the rind is pressed with a sponge, which absorbs the oil and is then squeezed out over a container, where it separates from any water or juices. Another method of extraction involves puncturing or pricking the rind to release the oil.

With solvent extraction, solvents such as petroleum ether, methanol, ethanol, or hexane are used to help bring oils in more fragile plants, including jasmine, gardenia, narcissus, neroli, and others.

The way CO_2 hypercritical extraction works is that CO_2 under high pressure will turn into a liquid. What's interesting about this method is that the process sometimes creates benefits for the oils that are not otherwise apparent. Frankincense and ginger are the most common essential oils extracted using this method.

Aromatherapy works because fragrance directly affects our body and our consciousness. As soon as you inhale any type of aroma, it will go straight to your brain, activating your limbic system where all emotions, memories, and behaviors live and are controlled. Endocrine glands are enhanced here as well. These glands regulates hormonal balance and make our body to work properly.

How the oils come to be, how people came to use them, and why they work, however, is not as important as how they are used. In the next chapters, we'll explore many popular oils and their benefits.

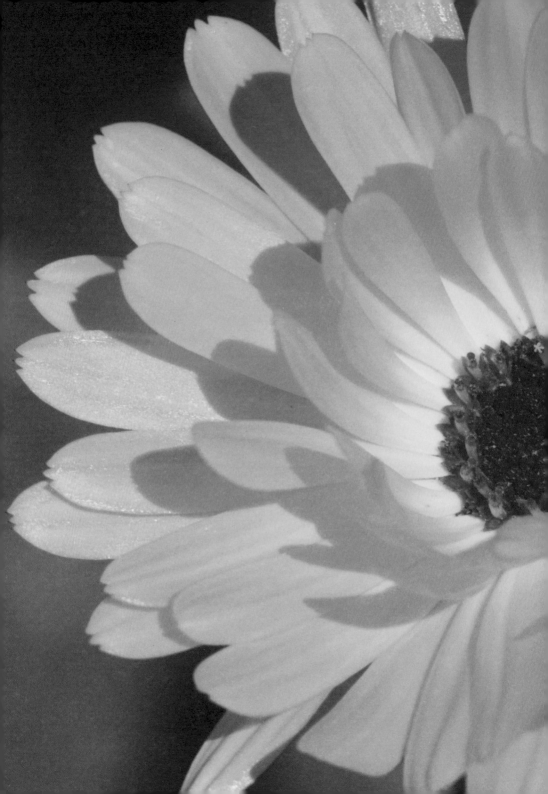

Carrier Oils

Carrier oils, also known as base oils, are used to dilute more concentrated essential oils. They are called carrier oils basically because they help "carry" essential oils to the places where they need to take effect. Carrier oils are generally pressed from seeds, nuts, and kernels, while essential oils are extracted from leaves, bark, and roots. Carrier oils have a shelf life, while essential oils do not. They may oxidize, thus losing some of their benefits, but they don't become rancid like carrier oils.

Like the choice of essential oil, which we'll get into in a bit, the choice of carrier oil will affect how your aromatics work. For now, let's look at some the most popular carrier oils.

Sweet Almond Oil

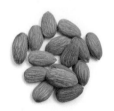

Sweet almond oil is light, slightly sweet, and absorbs well. Because it is warming, it makes for a great base for massage oil, especially when it comes to soothing joint and muscle pain. It's combined often with cinnamon and clove essential oils for this purpose. It's also used frequently to relieve itchy, dry skin.

Apricot Kernel Oil

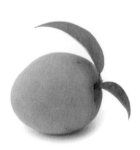

Apricot kernel is also widely used for massage. With a faint aroma and fairly quick absorption, it is warming and moisturizing. Because it is high in vitamin A and various minerals, it's also a boon to the skin. It is used for moisturizing but also for respiratory and digestive issues, often used in combination with eucalyptus or peppermint oil for respiratory issues and on its own for digestive issues.

ARNICA OIL

Arnica has been widely used for medically since the fifteenth century to treat a wide range of ailments, from arthritis to bruises and insect bites, as well as helping get rid of boils, acne, and other skin conditions. It's most effective when applied directly to the affected area. Long ago, the dried leaves of the plant would be smoked to treat coughs and colds, but that hasn't been in practice for a good many years. In the 1980s, arnica was analyzed by German scientists who discovered that it actually contained key compounds proven to reduce pain and inflammation.

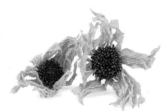

AVOCADO OIL

An extremely moisturizing oil, avocado oil is very strong and needs to be used sparingly with essential oils, as it does have a tendency to overpower other oils. It's generally used for its cooling and calming qualities, and is often used in combination with chamomile or lavender essential oils as a massage oil to

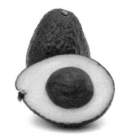

help ease symptoms of PMS or as a relaxant to improve sleep. High in vitamin E and monounsaturated fats, it's also frequently used in skin care products.

BORAGE SEED OIL

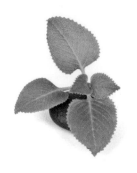

Borage seed oil has been studied for treatment of various ailments including inflammation, arthritis, and skin disorders including eczema, as well as for treating stress, PMS, ADHD, and alcoholism. On the downside, excessive use of borage oil has been shown to lead to liver disease, promote seizures, and may not be safe during pregnancy, as it can possibly trigger premature labor.

CALENDULA OIL

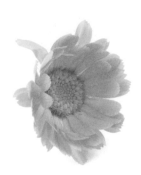

Calendula is a soothing, quick-absorbing oil used to treat spider veins, varicose veins, and leg ulcers. It is good for use on sensitive skin and has an antiseptic quality that makes it good for treating diaper rashes and other skin conditions, including eczema, dermatitis, psoriasis. It's anti-fungal, which helps treat conditions like jock itch, ringworm, and athlete's foot. It's antimicrobial, which helps heal mild cuts, bed sores, acne, and insect bites, and also helps prevents scarring.

Cedarwood Oil

Cedarwood is a repellent of bedbugs and mites. It is a sedative, too, when applied to the base of the neck. It is **never** taken internally.

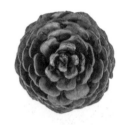

Evening Primrose Oil

A light, sweet oil, evening primrose is mostly used in treating skin conditions, including psoriasis, eczema, as well as to purify the blood and blood and to improve sexual energies when combined with vanilla or ylang ylang oils.

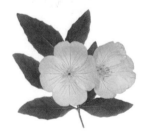

Grapeseed Oil

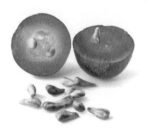

Grapeseed oil is a purifying antioxidant good for removing toxins and cleansing when mixed with tee tree oil. It makes a good lubricant for shaving and is also used as a growth stimulant and strengthener for hair.

Jojoba Oil

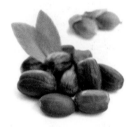

While jojoba oil is technically a wax, and it tends to be expensive, not as much of it is required as with other types of oils. Because it is a light, silky oil that absorbs well, it's great for the skin and good for treating acne, psoriasis, and atopic dermatitis as it doesn't block pores. It also great for nails, especially the cuticles, and hair. It makes a wonderful pre-shampooing conditioner when applied at least an hour before shampooing to treat scalp and hair follicles—only a few drops are needed.

Rosehip Seed Oil

A light, mild, clear oil, rosehip seed oil is used to treat skin conditions, and combines well with bergamot and grapefruit oils for nourishing skin and soothing inflammation.

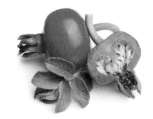

Seabuckthorn Berry Oil

Rich in essential fatty acids, vitamins, minerals and other nutrients, seabuckthorn oil is generally used as an anti-inflammatory and to soothe sun damage, as well as to heal wounds.

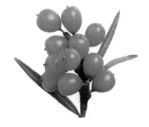

Sesame Oil

Because it's thick and oily, sesame oil is not generally used as a massage oil carrier, but it does blend nicely with sweet-scented essential oils like vanilla and clove. While it can be soothing to dry skin and good for nails, it is also good for hair and scalp massage.

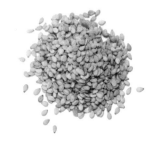

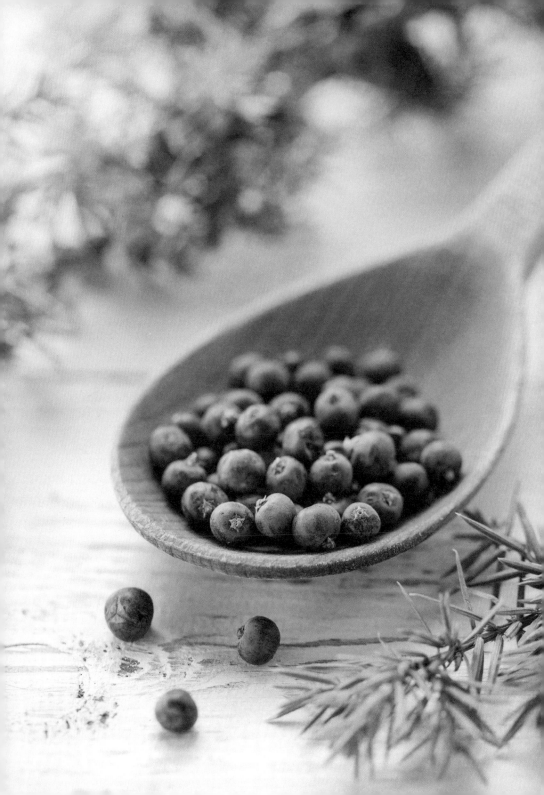

Essential Oils

The term "essential oil" is derived from the term "quintessential oil," and the concept dates back to ancient times when "quintessence," or spirit / life force, was considered the fifth element after fire, water, air, and earth. The ancients believed the practice of extracting these oils from plants was actually the removal of the spirit of the plant, hence the name.

Essential oils are not necessarily oils, but like oils, they are not water-soluble. Typically, they can be comprised of hundreds of aroma compounds. There are more than ninety essential oils, and each has its own health benefits. Most essential oils will benefit the body by cleaning receptor sites and returning cells to their healthiest state. They all help cells to regenerate and be protected. Some, however, have very specific characteristics for detailed uses, so if you have to have one or other oils, choose from the following selection.

Basil Oil

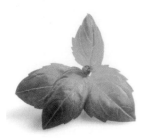

Basil oil is used to treat digestive issues like nausea, indigestion, and constipation, as well as motion sickness and respiratory problems. The ancients also used basil oil to treat colds, infections, and for skin care. It blends well with bergamot, clary sage, clove bud, geranium, lime, lemon, hyssop, juniper, eucalyptus, neroli, marjoram, rosemary, and lavender.

Bay Oil

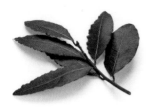

Bay oil has been used as a pain reliever, appetite stimulant, fever reducer, spasm controller, and even to stop hair loss. It is also widely believed to eliminate toxins and calm nervous afflictions.

Bergamot Oil

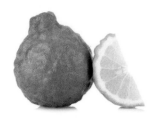

Bergamot oil has many uses, from suppressing pain to healing cuts and scars to improving digestion. It is also used as a mood-enhancer, a sleep aid, and as a deodorant.

Cardamon Oil

From enhancing libido to promoting respiratory health and reducing nausea, cardamon oil has many uses. Because it stimulates urination, it's also widely considered a detox oil.

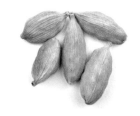

Carrot Seed Oil

Carrot seed oil is used to fight infections and also helps to remove excess gas from the body as well as other detoxifying measures. It is also known to promote cell regeneration.

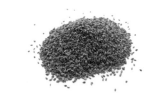

Cinnamon Oil

Cinnamon oil does more than eliminate bad breath. It is also used to treat infections, heal wounds, and relieve pain.

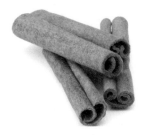

Clary Sage Oil

An antidepressant, clary sage essential oil is said to fight depression, manage anxiety, and uplift mood, as well as decrease sexual dysfunction and increase libido.

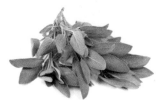

CLOVE OIL

Clove oil is great for dental issues, including toothaches and cavities but has also shown to be useful in treating many ailments, including infections and headaches. It's also been used to strengthen the immune system and to treat nausea, indigestion, and even premature ejaculation.

EUCALYPTUS OIL

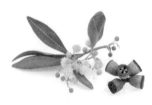

While it's used often in treating respiratory problems, eucalyptus oil is also used to relieve muscle pain and intestinal discomfort, for dental issues, and to ease exhaustion.

FENNEL OIL

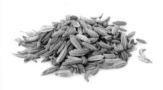

Fennel oil aids in digestion by increasing appetite and helping relieve excess gas and constipation, but also defends against colds and helps decrease infection.

Frankincense Oil

Frankincense is an astringent that helps fight infections, promotes immunity, heals scars, helps in cell regeneration, and soothes anxiety. It reduces inflammation, purifies the system, and helps make the body alkaline. It is one of the **must haves** in your set.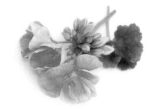

Geranium Oil

Geranium oil is mainly used to help stop hemorrhaging but is also used to kill intestinal parasites as well as to prevent body odor.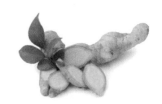

Ginger Oil

Ginger oil combats nausea and is known to improve brain and memory function, as well as to break fevers, improve stomach health, and detox the body.

Grapefruit Oil

Used to stimulate urination and fight infections, grapefruit oil is also helpful in reducing depression and mood enhancement.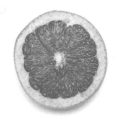

Juniper Berry Oil

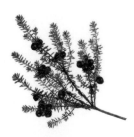

Juniper essential oil has been used to treat rheumatism and arthritis, to stop hemorrhaging and to help heal wounds.

Lavender Oil

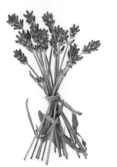

Lavender oil is calming and has been known to help with insomnia, but it also aids in digestion and immunity. This is another **must have**. It is a natural antihistamine, great for cat allergies, drying wounds, any skin ailment, and for relaxation.

Lemon Oil

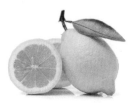

In addition to warding off infection, lemon oil is known to firm muscles and skin, strengthen the gums, and even combat hair loss.

Lemongrass Oil

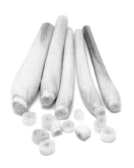

Lemongrass oil is known to reduce pain, but it also lifts depression, reduces body odor, and soothes inflammation. It is considered a "hot oil," meaning that applying directly onto the skin may cause some irritation or a sense of extreme warmth.

MELALEUCA OR TEA TREE OIL

Tea tree essential oil is essentially used to keep infection at bay and eradicate coughs and colds, but it also helps speed healing and prevent scarring.

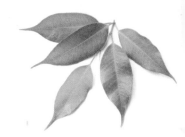

MAY CHANG "MOUNTAIN PEPPER" OIL

May chang essential oil relieves fatigue and tempers anxiety and stress. It's helpful in the treatment of acne and oily skin, and is used as a deodorant in lotions. It has a "citrusy" quality and blends with many other oils, including basil, bergamot, clary sage, geranium, ginger, jasmine, lavender, rosemary, and ylang ylang.

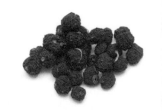

MELISSA OIL (LEMON BALM)

Melissa oil is commonly used to temper depression, but it's also good for lowering blood pressure, treating fever, boosting immunity, and helping digestion.

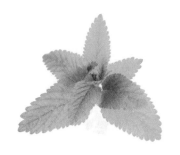

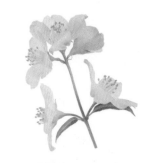

Neroli Oil

Neroli essential oil is a famous aphrodisiac but it's also a mood enhancer, anxiety soother, and reduces inflammation and helps reduce scarring in healing.

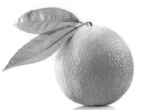

Orange Oil

Orange essential oil is great for uplifting your mood and soothing anxiety, and is useful in allieviating sexual dysfunction.

Palmarosa Oil

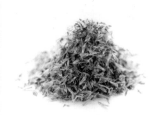

Palmarosa oil (also known as Indian or Turkish geranium oil) comes from Ethiopia, and is great for skin health due to its moisturizing properties. It nourishes and restores both oily and dry skin. (Note: Avoid using during pregnancy.)

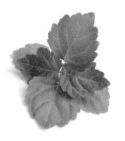

Patchouli Oil

Patchouli oil is used to fight depression but also has strong physical properties, including helping to cure fever and kill fungal issues.

Peppermint Oil

Peppermint oil relieves occasional stomach and intestinal discomfort because of its active ingredient menthol.

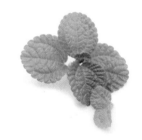

Pine Oil

Pine oil is good for the skin but also helps increase metabolism, relieve pain relief, and is useful in treating urinary tract infections and respiratory problems.

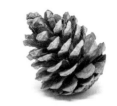

Ravensara Oil

Native to the island of Madagascar and used for centuries for fighting infections, ravensara oil has powerful properties and is good for shingles, cold sores, achy muscles, bacterial infections, colds, respiratory problems, and pain relief. It blends well with many oils, such as frankincense, tea tree, rosemary, thyme, eucalyptus, geranium, lavender, and lemon. (Note: Avoid use during pregnancy.)

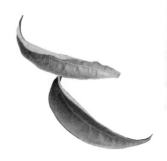

ROMAN CHAMOMILE OIL

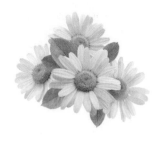

Roman chamomile essential oil is popular and useful for physical and emotional conditions. Physically, it aids in digestion and helps cure pain, and is widely used to temper fever. It's also good for the liver. Emotionally, it's used to fight depression and uplift mood.

ROSE OIL

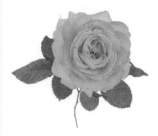

Rose essential oil has works as a laxative, among other benefits, and fights depression and enhances libido.

ROSEMARY OIL

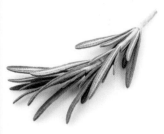

Rosemary essential oil is often used for hair and skin care, but is also useful for treating gums. It's helpful in treating anxiety and depression and is a mood enhancer. It also aids in digestion and helps temper indigestion and flatulence, among other benefits.

SANDALWOOD OIL

Sandalwood essential oil has many physical benefits, including boosting immunity, protecting against infection, soothing inflammation, stopping hemorrhaging, and preventing hair loss.

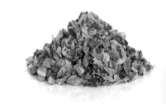

SAVORY OIL

Savory oil is strongly antiseptic and helps prevent scarring. It's used mainly for treating bites, burns, ulcers, and abscesses.

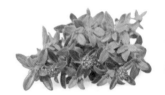

SPRUCE OIL

Spruce oil is frequently used as a disinfectant but also has physical and emotional health benefits, including fighting infection, boosting immunity, and for easing aches and pains and relieving asthma and bronchitis. It's been used to combat fatigue, to soothe skin conditions, to fight fungal infections, to ease muscle pain, and also to ward against scarring.

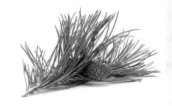

Star Anise Oil

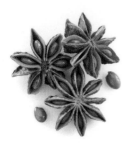

Star Anise oil has a strong aroma reminiscent of black licorice and can be used to help ease bronchitis, colds, and the flu, as well as in adding digestion and soothing muscular aches or pains.

Vanilla Oil

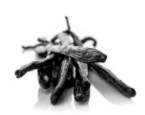

Vanilla essential oil is a known aphrodisiac but it also has many health benefits, including reducing fever, and inflammation. For balance and well-being, it is used for hormone balance and alleviating depression. It is also effective as an antioxidant and antibacterial.

Vetiver Oil

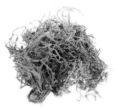
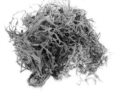

Vetiver essential oil is generally used to soothe inflammation, boost immunity, enhance libido, and to prevent scarring.

Ylang Ylang Oil

Ylang ylang oil is used to combat depression and as a mood enhancer but is also used for reducing blood pressure.

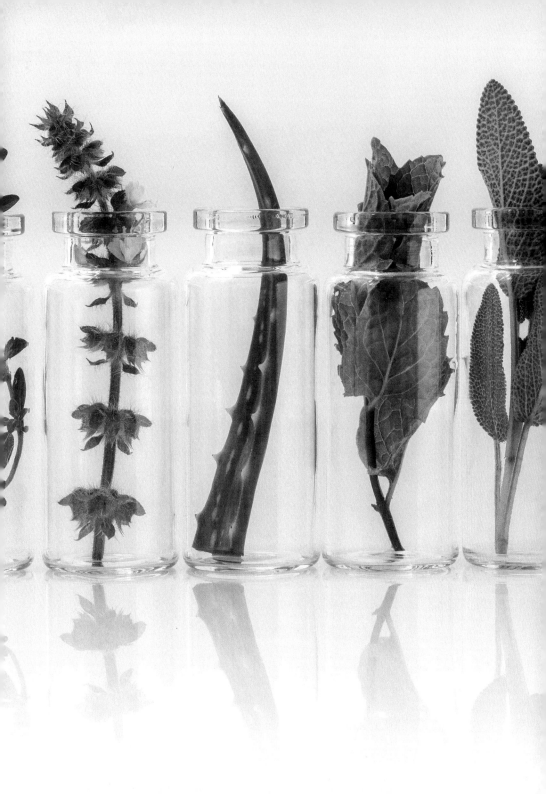

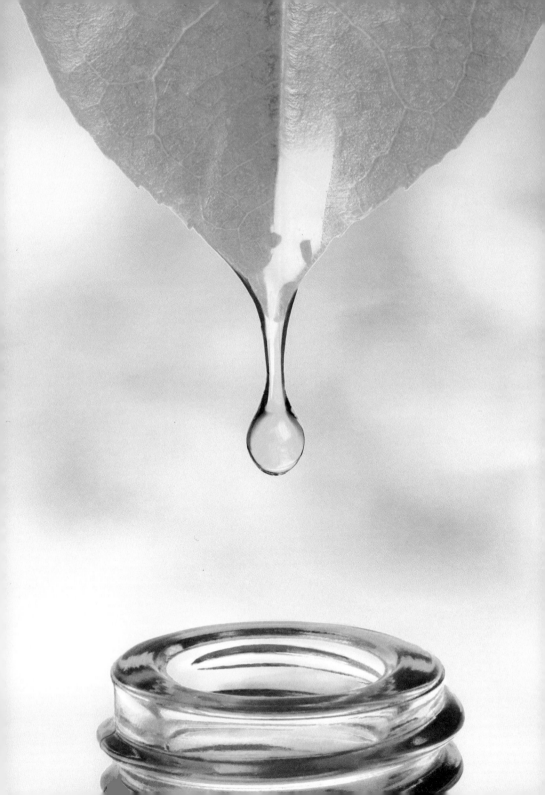

Recipes

*n*ow that you know all about the different aromatherapy components, it's time to start "cooking."
In this section, we'll cover many ways you can use
combinations of essential oils to enhance your physical,
mental, and emotional well-being. From increasing energy,
boosting immunity, relieving headaches, and staying calm
to keeping a fresh-smelling home, there is an oil recipe for
every need—even some for pets!

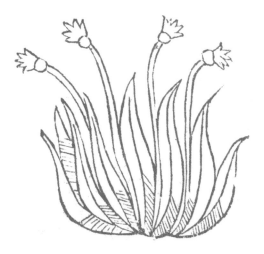

Balance Equilibrium

It doesn't take long before everyday stress begins to wear us down. Balancing family, work, and relationships takes energy. These recipes are designed to bring you back to a calm, peaceful, and balanced state. With more energy and less stress, you will be able to confront all of life's challenges with improved concentration and focus.

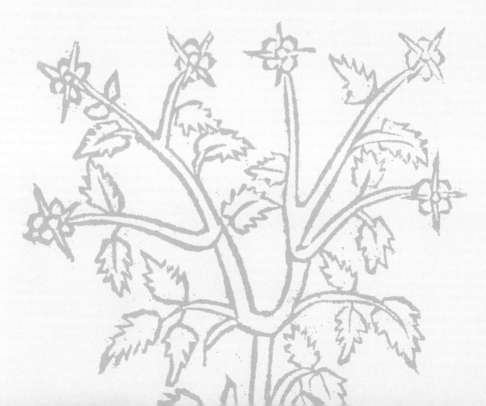

Depression

Most people deal with some form of depression throughout their lives. Use this recipe to increase your vitality to ward off the blues.

Combine:

4 drops lavender

3 drops clary sage

2 drops ylang ylang

1 drop marjoram

How to Use:

Add to your diffuser, following manufacturer's instructions.

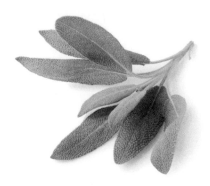

Mood

After showering, you can rub 4 drops of this combination into your wet hair. Capture the aroma in your hands; the vapors fill the air and will enhance your mood while softening your hair.

4 drops lavender

2 drops cedarwood

2 drops orange

1 drop ylang ylang

1 drop vetiver

How to Use:

Add to your diffuser, following manufacturer's instructions.

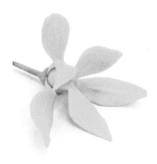

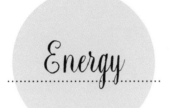

Energy

Need some pep in your step? This will lift the spirit and wake up the brain.

Combine:
4 drops wild orange
4 drops peppermint

How to Use:
Add to your diffuser, following manufacturer's instructions.

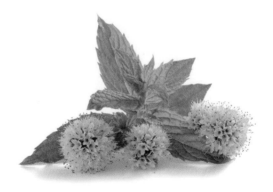

Stress Relief

Calms the furious, diminishes anger, and replaces negative thoughts. Roman chamomile can have a strong smell so apply this away from your nose.

Combine:

4 drops Roman chamomile

3 drops lavender

2 drops clary sage

2 drops geranium

1 drop ylang ylang

How to Use:

Add to your diffuser, following manufacturer's instructions.

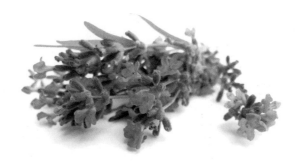

Weight Loss

Use to encourage healthy digestion and to speed up metabolism.

Combine:

15 drops basil

15 drops marjoram

1 drop oregano

1 drop thyme

How to Use:

Add to your diffuser, following manufacturer's instructions.

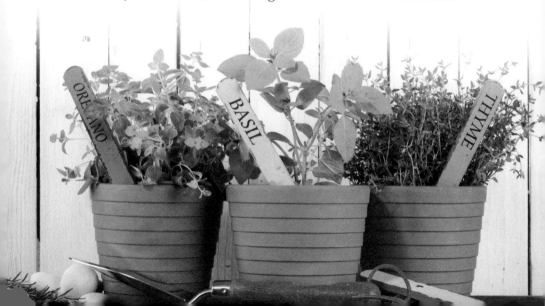

Balancing Bath Oil

For any time of day or night, this bath will calm and relax
your mind while elevating your spirits.

Combine:

30 drops sandalwood

12 drops lavender

2 drops cedarwood

Then Add:

4fl oz (125ml) of carrier oil of your choice, such as jojoba or
   sweet almond oil

How to Use:

Combine all the ingredients in a dark glass or plastic bottle.
Store it in a cool, dark place, and when ready, pour a
tablespoon into bathwater.

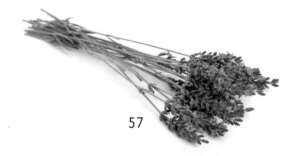

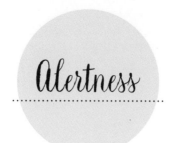

Alertness

Removing blockages can help stimulate thought and clarity.

Combine:

2 drops wild orange

2 drops bergamot

2 drops cypress

2 drops frankincense

How to Use:

Add to your diffuser, following manufacturer's instructions.

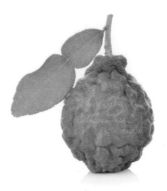

Clarity

This blend can aid meditation and induce thoughtfulness.

Combine:

2 drops orange

2 drops peppermint

How to Use:

Add to your diffuser, following manufacturer's instructions.

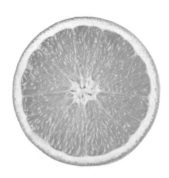

Concentration

When you've got to put in the hours, this will give you the power.

Combine:
1 drop basil
2 drops rosemary
2 drops cypress

Then Add:
¼ C (60ml) carrier oil, such as apricot or jojoba

How to Use:
Combine all ingredients and use either in a room diffuser, air freshener, or by misting with a spray bottle.

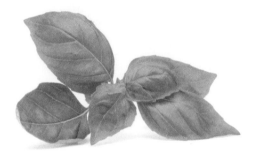

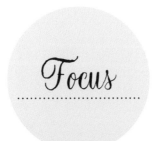

Focus

This combination will allow you to stay on track and keep your eye trained on what is important.

Combine:

6 drops ginger

5 drops grapefruit

4 drops juniper berry

Then add:

15 ml carrier oil

How to Use:

Combine essential oils with carrier oil and use for massage.

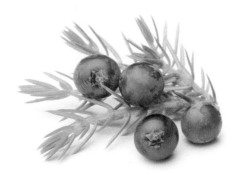

Memory

Helps clear your body from heavy metal toxicity and also will aid concentration, alertness, and relieve anxiety.

Combine:

4 drops basil

8 drops rosemary

8 drops cypress

How to Use:

Add to your diffuser, following manufacturer's instructions.

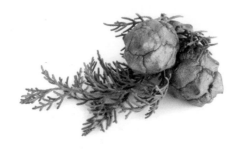

Relaxing Bath Oil

Reduces inflammation, purifies the system, and flushes acidity from your system; one of the "must have" oil combinations in your life.

Combine:
10 drops lavender
5 drops frankincense
5 drops marjoram
1 drop cedarwood

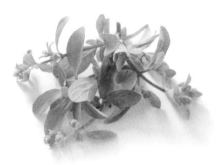

Then add:
4fl oz (125ml) of carrier oil of your choice, such as jojoba or sweet almond oil

How to Use:
Combine all the ingredients in a dark glass or plastic bottle. Store it in a cool, dark place and, when ready, pour a tablespoon into bathwater.

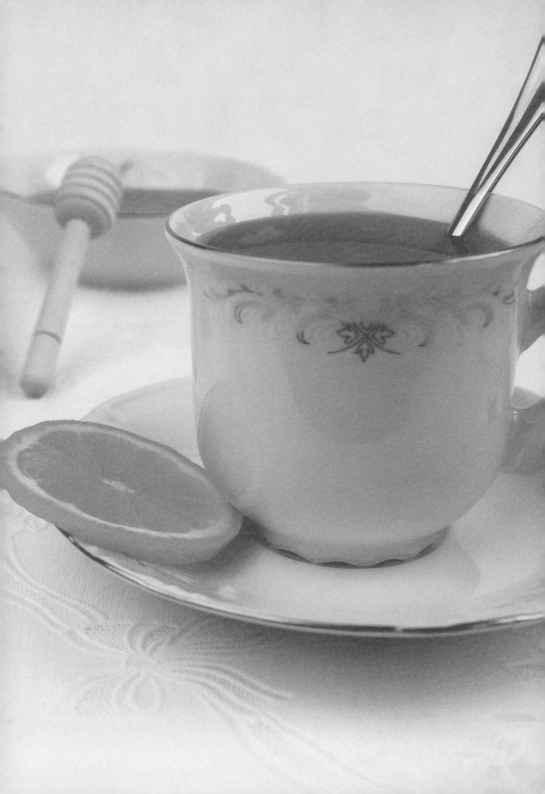

Fight Sickness

No matter how hard we try to keep ourselves healthy, it is inevitable that a cold will strike. The oils here will boost your immunity against colds and coughs, congestion, and respiratory problems, or will help relieve already-present symptoms.

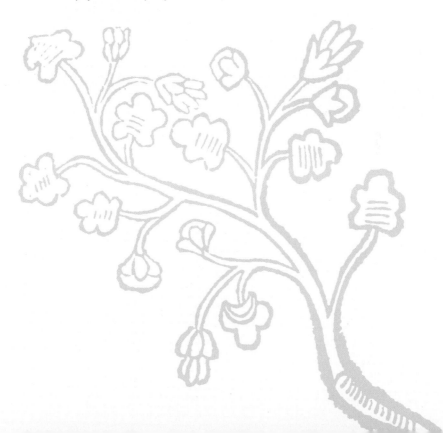

Immunity

Your immune system is the most important defender of your body from disease.

Combine:

5 drops lavender

5 drops eucalyptus

3 drops ravensara

2 drops bay laurel

How to Use:

Add to your diffuser, following manufacturer's instructions.

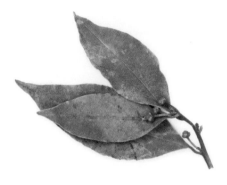

Colds & Coughs

Excellent for draining nasal and chest cavities, and for stimulating blood flow.

Combine:

6 drops cinnamon

6 drops rosemary

6 drops pine

3 drops thyme

Then add:

5 drops per 18 ounces of hot water.

How to Use:

Add to your diffuser, following manufacturer's instructions.

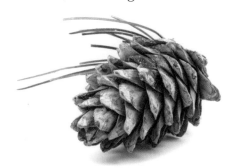

Congestion

An anti-rheumatic remedy to sooth and assist with breathing.

Combine:

20 drops orange

10 drops eucalyptus

10 drops juniper berry

10 drops pine

6 drops basil

6 drops rosewood

4 drops ginger

How to Use:

Add to your diffuser, following manufacturer's instructions.

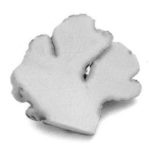

Respiratory System

This is great for the cardiovascular and pulmonary system, as well as a real wake-up call for the lungs.

Combine:
1 drop lemon

1 drop lime

1 drop peppermint

1 drop rosemary

1 drop eucalyptus

How to Use:
Add to your diffuser, following manufacturer's instructions.

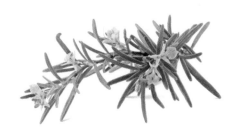

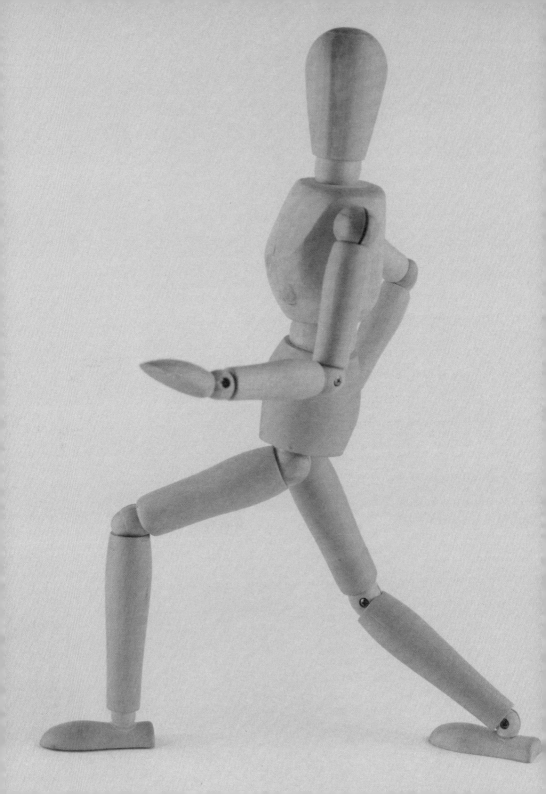

Stop Pain & Strain

Nothing is more frustrating than pain, which hinders our balanced state and makes our body and mind misaligned. Whether it stems from working out, headaches, or menstrual cycles, these combinations not only act as natural healing remedies, but also invigorate the body.

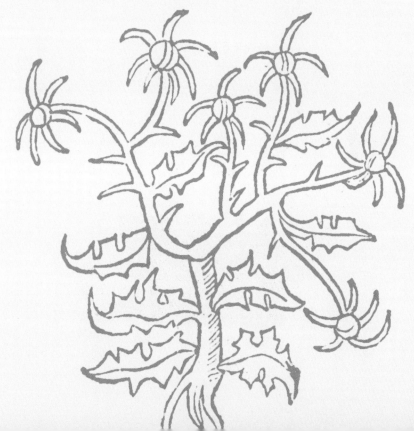

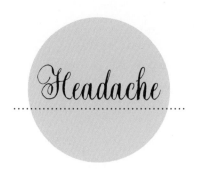

Headache

To relieve or ease pain, try 2 drops of this combination near your temples.

Combine:
5 drops marjoram
5 drops thyme
5 drops rosemary
5 drops peppermint
5 drops lavender

How to Use:
Add to diffuser following manufacturer's instructions and keep diffuser close to you head.

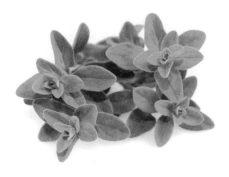

Joint Pain

This recipe will drive away aches and invigorate, while reducing swelling of the joints.

Combine:
10 drops marjoram
8 drops eucalyptus
4 drops cajuput
2 drops black pepper

Then add:
1 cup carrier oil

How to Use:
Add carrier oil and essential oils to a jar, close lid, and shake well. Rub onto sore joints.

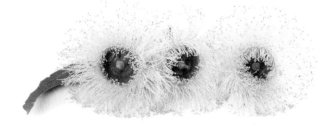

Muscle Pain

If pain creeps in before (or after) a work out, this makes for a great body rub.

Combine:
20 drops ylang ylang
20 drops ginger
12 drops nutmeg
8 drops rosemary

Then add:
2 ounces almond oil

How to Use:
Blend essential oils with almond carrier oil and warm slightly. Massage onto sore muscles.

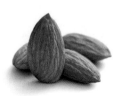

Menstrual Cramps

Reduce muscle tension to allow your lower torso to expand and relax.

Combine:

10 drops rose

7 drops roman chamomile

7 drops geranium

7 drops lavender

4 drops clary sage

Then add:

30 ml jojoba oil

How to Use:

Blend essential oils with jojoba carrier oil and massage onto lower back at least once a day while symptoms ensue.

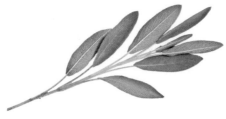

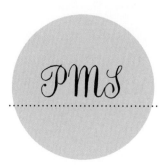

PMS

Regulating moods can be a huge help during monthly cycles, so keep this on hand.

Combine:
5 drops rose
12 drops clary sage
9 drops bergamot

How to Use:
Blend oils and add 5–7 drops into bath water.

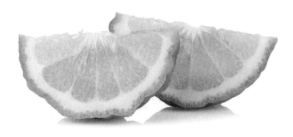

Muscle Energizer Bath

Soothe and revitalize skin and muscles with this easy bath remedy.

Combine:

2 drops eucalyptus or rosemary

1 drop palmarosa

1 drop peppermint

How to Use:

Combine the ingredients directly into a bath with two cups of dissolved epsom salt. (Note: **Do not** use this recipe if you have high blood pressure.)

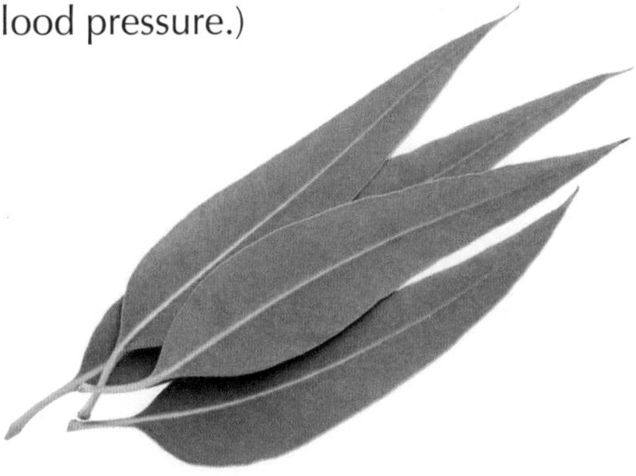

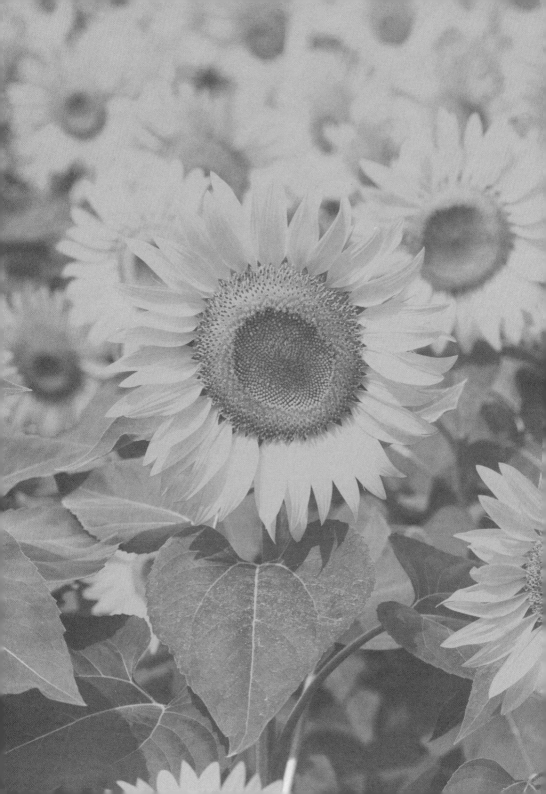

Feel Better

llergies, nausea, and upset stomachs are those annoying little things that seem to pop up out of nowhere, and can quickly escalate to make you feel just plain awful. In this section we use oils that will make you feel better and more complete.

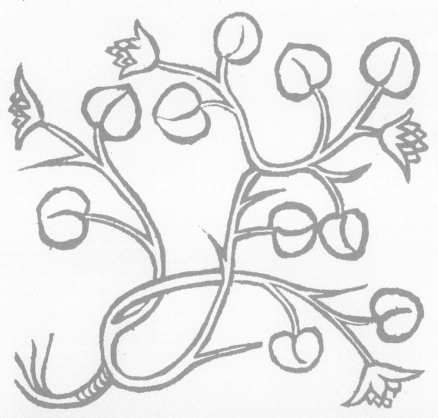

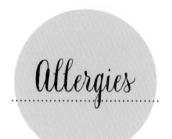

Allergies

Clear permanent sinusitis with a home-made mixture. Mix 2 drops of each of the oils to a small container with hot water. Close your eyes and inhale deeply.

Combine:

2 drops peppermint

2 drops lemon

2 drops lavender

How to Use:

Add to your diffuser.

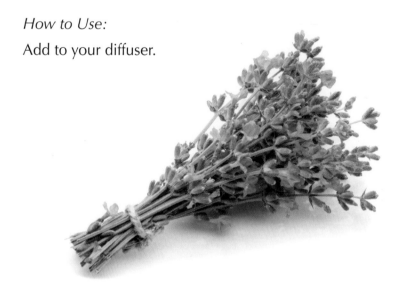

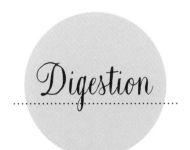

Digestion

The best way to clear negative thinking is by cleaning your intestinal system.

Combine:

5 drops bergamot

3 drops ginger

3 drops Roman chamomile

Then add:

1 ounce grapeseed oil

How to Use:

Combine essential with grapeseed carrier oil. Massage over stomach and intestinal areas.

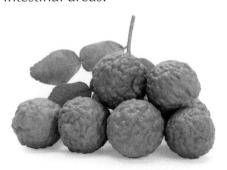

Motion Sickness

Motion sickness is sometimes referred to as sea sickness or car sickness, and can happen from any kind of movement, even movement you are anticipating.

Combine:
4 drops nutmeg

6 drops tangerine

3 drops Roman chamomile

2 drops cardamon

How to Use:
Add a couple of drops to a cotton ball and inhale when needed.

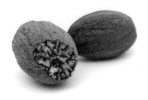

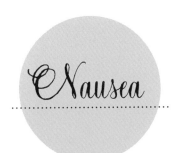

Nausea

Use this to keep your stomach in check. (Note: If nausea is prolonged, see your doctor.)

Combine:
1 drop basil
1 drop peppermint
1 drop lavender

Then add:
2 teaspoons grapeseed oil

How to Use:
Combine oils and warm by rubbing mixture between your palms. Apply over your stomach.

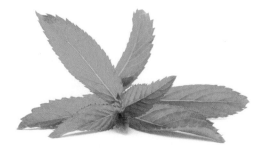

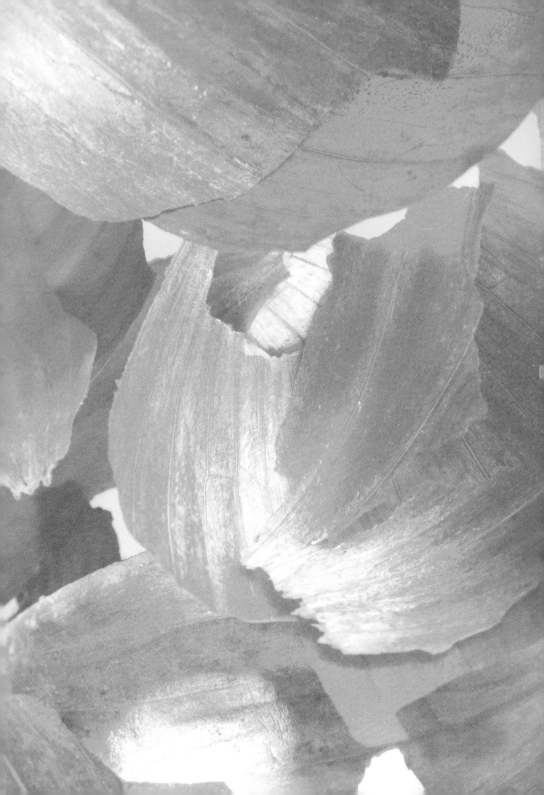

Help for the Skin

Skin irritations can be unsightly, not to mention frustrating and uncomfortable. As an alternative to harsh treatments, use these natural recipes as a daily cleansing routine or to soothe bug bites, burns, and bruises.

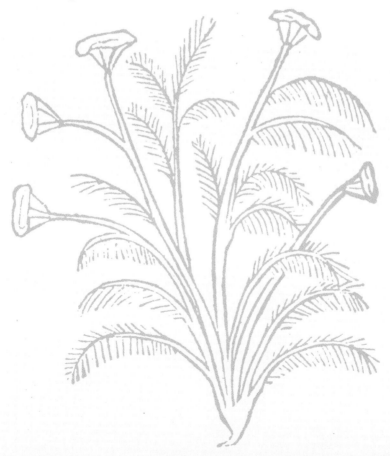

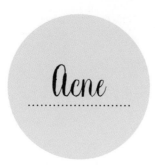

Acne

This help's dry wounds and is great for any skin ailment.

Combine:

8 drops lavender

4 drops tea tree

Then add:

½ ounce kukui nut oil

3 drops cypress oil

2 drops helichrysum

How to Use:

Combine essential oils with kukui nut carrier oil. Apply to affected area several times per day.

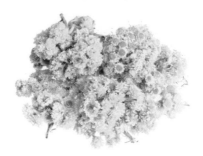

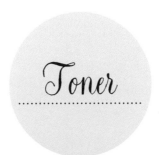

Toner

Use this natural toner as an essential part of your daily cleansing routine for a healthy face.

Combine:

2 drops lavender

1 drop palmarosa

1 drop rosewood

How to Use:

Apply on a clean face with cotton ball before foundation for daytime and at night before bed.

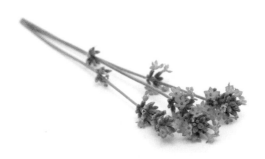

Bug Bites

Reduces irritation and soothing to the skin. (Note: It may have a strong scent.)

Combine:

2 drops Roman chamomile

3 drops eucalyptus

3 drops lavender

1 drop peppermint

Then add:

1 ounce cider vinegar

How to Use:

Blend oils with cider vinegar and apply to affected area with cotton ball several times a day, as needed.

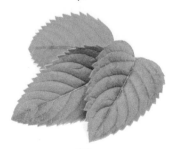

Burns & Bruises

To cleanse, calm, and condition, this recipe also encourages regrowth of the skin.

Combine:

4 drops Roman chamomile

6 drops geranium

6 drops lavender

4 drops lemon

2 drops tea tree

How to Use:

Blend oils together and add several drops to a basin of warm water. Apply to affected area with a soft cloth.

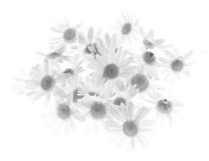

Get Some Rest

Sleep is vital for good health, as it allows our minds and bodies to rest and heal. It doesn't take much for our internal sleep rhythm to get out of whack from stress and worry. Here are a couple of mixtures to help you fall asleep and stay asleep—as well as a couple for other bedroom activities.

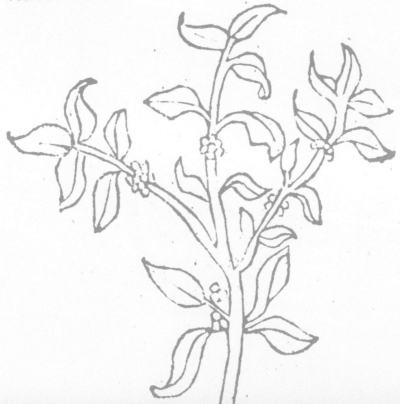

Falling Asleep

When you want to drop off to slumber without the toss and turn, use this soothing mixture.

Combine:
6 drops grapefruit
6 drops bergamot
6 drops lime
4 drops ginger
2 drops sandalwood

How to Use:
Add to your diffuser, following manufacturer's instructions.

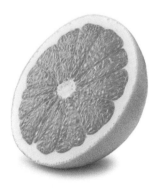

Staying Asleep

Use this floral mixture for restive sleep with happy dreams.

Combine:

8–10 drops lavender

2–3 drops palmarosa

2–3 drops rose geranium

How to Use:

Add to your diffuser, following manufacturer's instructions.

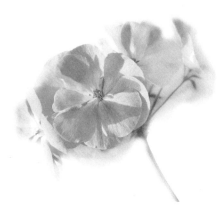

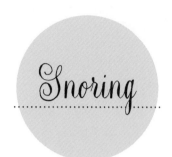

Snoring

If your partner's snoring keeps you awake, use this to give both of you a better night's sleep.

Combine:

9 drops lavender

4 drops marjoram

3 drops lemon

Then add:

¼ C (60ml) carrier oil, such as apricot or jojoba

How to Use:

Combine all ingredients in dark glass, and wait 24 hours after blending for the oil to cure. To use, rub the massage oil gently onto the upper chest, neck, and the bones behind the ears.

Sex Drive

A natutral remedy for when a little help is needed to move things along.

Combine:

7–10 drops sandalwood

2 drops vanilla

1 drop ylang ylang

How to Use:

Add to your diffuser, following manufacturer's instructions.

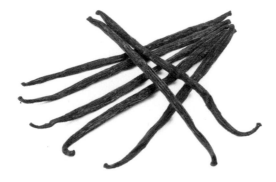

Sensual Massage Oil

To get in the mood, use this delightful external blend to soften muscles and excite the senses.

Combine:

8 drops sandalwood

3 drops orange

2 drops patchouli

1 drop ylang ylang

1 drop ginger

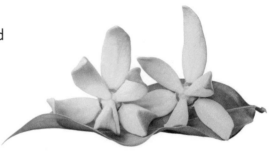

Then add:

¼ C (60ml) carrier oil such as apricot or jojoba

How to Use:

Combine all the ingredients in a dark glass or plastic bottle. Store it in a cool, dark place and, when ready, pour into a bottom with a spray or dispenser cap to control the oil flow.

Sweet Dreams Bath Oil

Be sure to get into bed before you head off to a deep sleep with this mixture.

Combine:

20 drops of lavender

16 drops of orange

4 drops clary sage

1 drop vitiver

1 drop ylang ylang

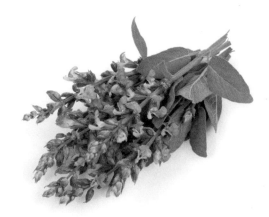

Then add:

4 fl oz (125ml) carrier oil

How to Use:

Combine all the ingredients in a dark glass or plastic bottle. Store it in a cool, dark place and, when ready, pour a tablespoon into bathwater.

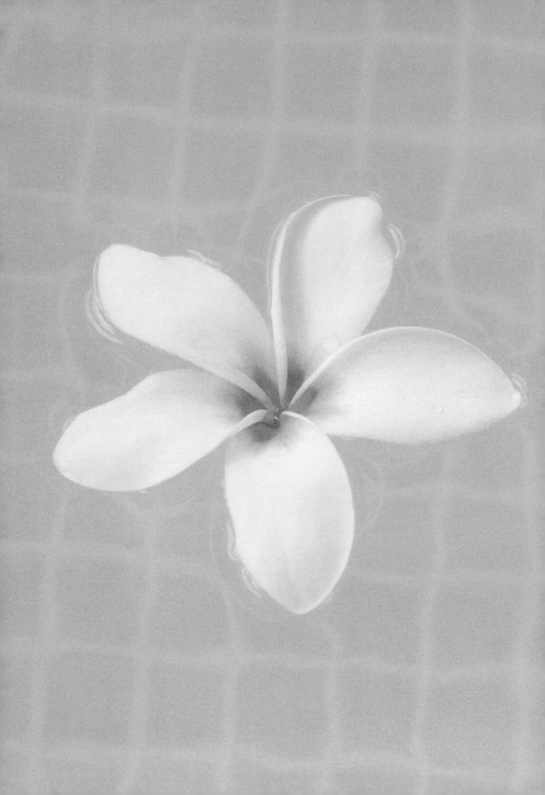

Enjoy a Spa Day

Who needs over-the-counter beauty products or expensive spas! Stay at home and pamper yourself with a spa day. From helping a pesky dry scalp to moisturizing your entire body and face, these luxurious recipes will make you feel brand new.

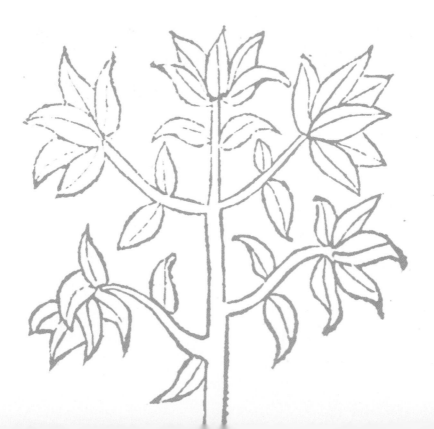

Body Moisturizer

Softening your skin helps to soften our thoughts and makes us feel great.

Combine:

25 drops carrot seed

6 drops sandalwood

4 drops neroli

2 drops geranium

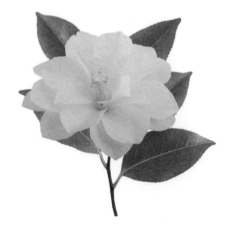

Then add:

1 teaspoon jojoba oil

1 teaspoon camelia oil

1 teaspoon sesame oil

How to Use:

Blend all ingredients and shake well. Apply to affected areas at least twice per day.

Face Moisturizer

A natural protector for the delicate skin on your face. Avoid placing on the eyes.

Combine:
1 drop geranium
2 drops lavender

Then add:
1 tablespoon almond oil

How to Use:
Combine oils and use on face after cleansing and toning.

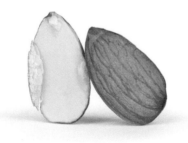

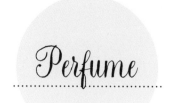

Perfume

Replace expensive perfumes with this delicious and natural blend of exotic oils.

Combine:
20 drops helichrysum
10 drops clary sage
10 drops bergamot
10 drops lavender
5 drops clove
5 drops rose otto
25 drops vanilla

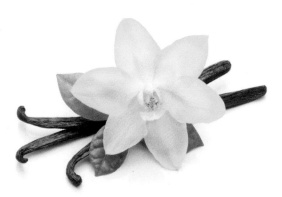

Then add:
1 ounce jojoba

How to Use:
Add vanilla to jojoba and then add the rest of the essential oils. Let sit for a week before using.

Scalp Treatment

For shiny hair and a healthy head, this also helps reduce dandruff.

Combine:
20 drops basil
10 drops cedarwood
10 drops rosemary

How to Use:
Blend oils and massage a few drops onto your scalp each night; shampoo in the morning.

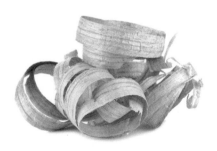

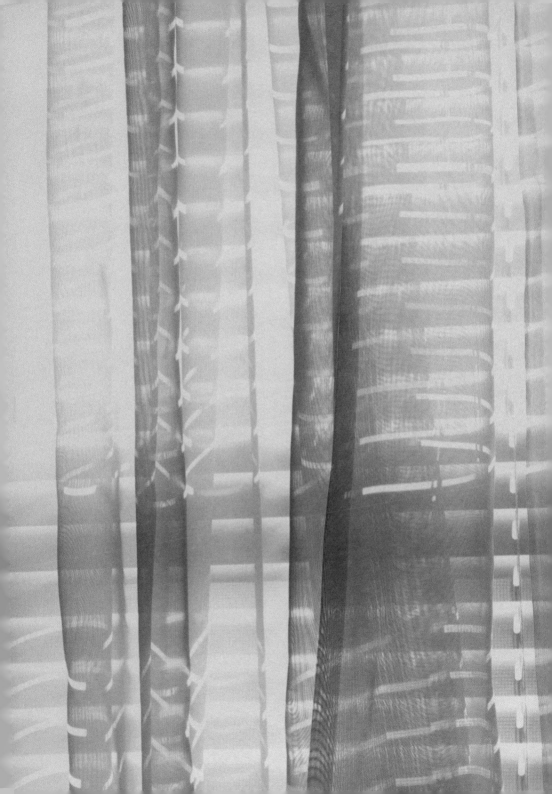

Freshen the Home

Essential oils not only work well on the body, but they are also ideal for the home, office, or car as disinfectants, cleaners, and air fresheners. With these natural mixtures, your home will always smell inviting and be clean year round!

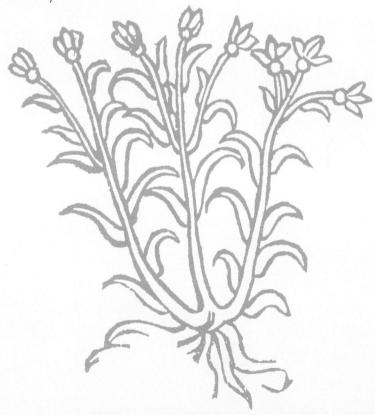

Carpet Freshener

Keep your home smelling fresh and inviting for when guests come over.

Combine:

30 drops eucalyptus

30 drops cinnamon

30 drops lemongrass

10 drops clove

Then add:

½ cup baking soda

How to Use:

Combine oils with baking soda in a jar. Let sit overnight or ideally for 1–2 days. Sprinkle over rug. Let sit 15 minutes then vacuum.

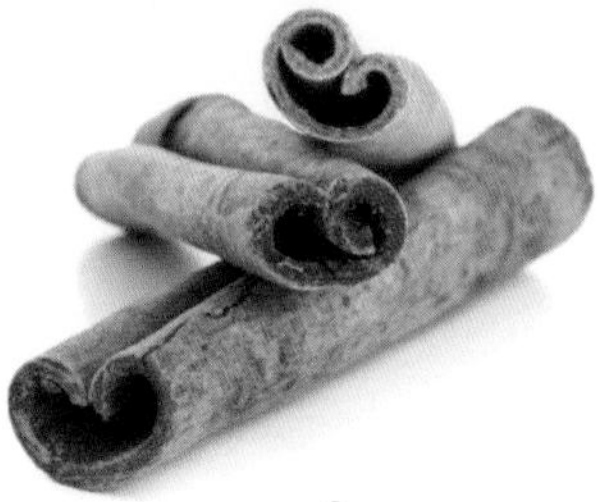

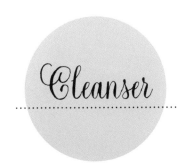

Cleanser

The natural way to keep your environment clean, fresh, and sweet-smelling.

Combine:
5 drops oregano
10 drops sage
10 drops thyme
20 drops lemon

Then add:
3 ml emulsifier
2 ½ cup distilled water

How to Use:
Add to spray bottle and shake well before using.

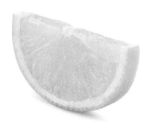

Disinfectant Spray

These natural astringents will make a safer environment for you, your family, and your pets.

Combine:
60 drops bergamot

40 drops oregano

25 drops spearmint

15 drops cedarwood

10 drops cinnamon

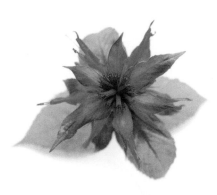

Then add:
5 ml emulsifier

4 ounces room spray base

How to Use:
Combine all ingredients into a spray bottle. Shake well before each use.

Glass Cleaner

Great for the car, office, bathroom mirror, or your eyeglasses.

Combine:

1 cup (250ml) water

1 cup (250ml) white vinegar

$1/4$ teaspoon (2ml) liquid dishwashing soap

5 drops lemon, tea tree, or lavender

How to Use:

To use, pour into a a spray bottle and shake well before using. Wipe off with newspaper or a lint-free cloth.

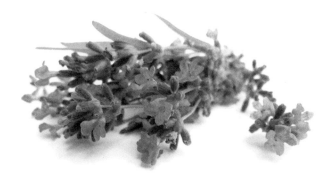

Fresh-Scent Deodorizer

For that new spring feeling all year round, this is like sunshine in a bottle.

Combine:

3 drops citronella

3 drops lavender

3 drops lemongrass

2 drops rosemary

2 drops myrtle

2 drops tea tree

¼ C (60ml) carrier oil,
    such as apricot or jojoba

How to Use:

Combine all the ingredients in a dark glass or plastic bottle. Store it in a cool, dark place, and, when ready, pour into a bottle with a spray/spritz cap to control the flow.

Spicy-Scent Deodorizer

Set a mood of excitement and action with this playful combination.

Combine:

3 drops cloves

3 drops lemon

3 drops cinnamon

2 drops eucalyptus

2 drops rosemary

Then add:

¼ C (60ml) carrier oil, such as apricot or jojoba

How to Use:

Combine all the ingredients in a dark glass or plastic bottle. Store it in a cool, dark place, and, when ready, pour into a bottle with a spray/spritz cap to control the flow.

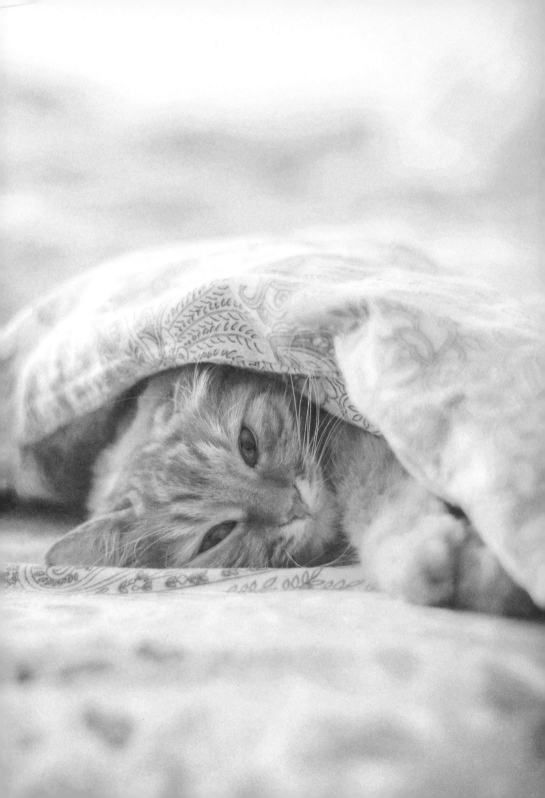

Pamper Your Pet

Our pets are a part of our families. Like humans, they, too, can benefit from essential oils for dry skin and insect repellent or as an odor refresher. Keep in mind that pets can be more sensitive than humans, so always use a mild, diluted solution on your pet, and be sure to do a spot test first.

Be very careful not to let the oils get near or in an animal's eyes. With cats, avoid high-phenol oils such as oregano and thyme, and felines are also typically ill-disposed to citrus. Use small doses (1 to 2 drops) for smaller animals, 3 to 4 drops for medium animals and 5 to 7 drops for larger animals, always diluted 80 to 90%

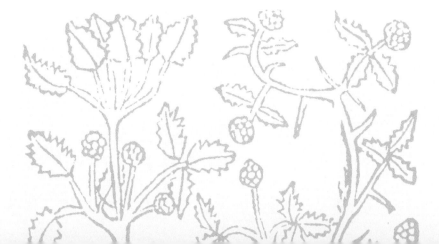

Dry Skin

Rub below the fur onto skin at the first sign of dry patches or scaly flakes.

Combine:

10 drops German chamomile

Then add:

1 tablespoon organic argan oil

How to Use:

Rub into affected area and cover for 15 to 20 minutes so pet can't lick it off.

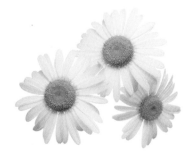

Flea Repellent

Repelling ticks and fleas is a must for any pet or owner who enjoys the outdoors.

Combine:
5 drops rosemary
5 drops peppermint
5 drops eucalyptus
5 drops tea tree
5 drops citronella

Then add:
1 cup purified water

How to Use:
Combine oils with water in a dark-colored spray bottle and shake well each time you use. Use every time you take your dog outside for a walk.

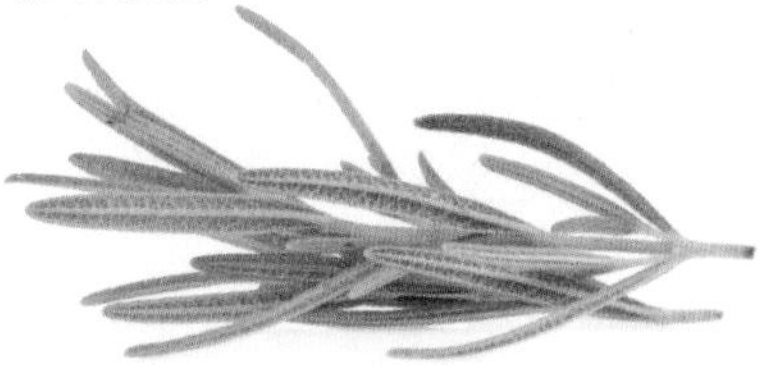

Insect Repellent

Keeping bugs at bay is important for all species.

Combine:

4–6 drops spearmint

3–5 drops peppermint

3–5 drops citronella

1 drop lemongrass

How to Use:

Add to your diffuser, following manufacturer's instructions.

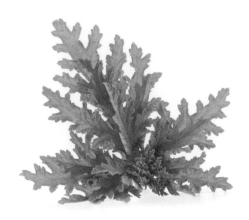

Pet Odor

Keep your house (and your dog) smelling fresh and inviting in between baths.

Combine:

10 drops orange

10 drops lavender

5 drops lemon

6 drops tea tree

5 drops geranium

2 drops nutmeg

3 drops neroli

How to Use:

Add 4–5 drops to diffuser, following manufacturer's instructions.

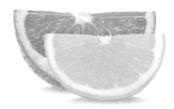

Anxiety

Thunder and lightning can be the cause of great anxiety for your dog or cat; this remedy can work for all anxious animals.

Combine:
2 drops ylang ylang
3 drops frankincense
2 drops rock rose

How to use:
Mix in a clean bowl and place 2 drops inside mouth, or on a cotton ball in front of the animals nose for inhaling.

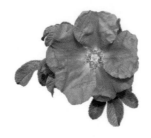

Photo Credits

Index